H. pylori Guide for Beginners

Symptoms and Complications of H. pylori Infection

By

Euan Kian

Table of Contents

CHAPTER 1
Introduction

1.1 What is H. pylori?

Helicobacter pylori, often abbreviated as H. pylori, is a type of bacteria that infects the human stomach and the upper part of the small intestine. It is a Gram-negative, spiral-shaped bacterium that can thrive in the acidic environment of the stomach, a place where most other bacteria cannot survive. Discovered in 1982 by Australian scientists Barry Marshall and Robin Warren, H. pylori has since been recognized as a significant factor in the development of various gastrointestinal diseases and has garnered substantial attention in the fields of medicine and microbiology.

H. pylori is a microorganism with a unique ability to colonize the mucous lining of the stomach, where it can persist for years or even decades if left untreated. This bacterium is highly adapted to its niche within the human body, as it has evolved several mechanisms to survive the harsh conditions of the stomach, such as the low pH (acidity) and the presence of gastric acids.

It's important to note that H. pylori infection is prevalent worldwide, with a higher incidence in developing countries. In some regions, a significant percentage of the population may carry the bacterium in their stomachs. While many individuals who are infected with H. pylori may remain asymptomatic, the presence of this bacterium has been strongly associated with the development of various gastrointestinal conditions, including:

- **Gastritis:** H. pylori infection can lead to inflammation of the stomach lining, known as gastritis. This inflammation can cause symptoms such as stomach pain, bloating, and nausea.

- **Peptic Ulcers:** One of the most well-known consequences of H. pylori infection is the development of peptic ulcers. These are soring that form in the lining of the stomach or the duodenum (the first part of the small intestine). They can be quite painful and lead to complications if left untreated.

- **Gastric Cancer:** H. pylori infection is a significant risk factor for the development of gastric (stomach) cancer. While not everyone with H. pylori will develop cancer, long-term infection can increase the likelihood of this serious condition.

Despite its association with various health problems, it's important to recognize that not everyone who carries H. pylori will experience these issues. The interplay between the bacterium, the host's genetics, and environmental factors plays a complex role in determining the outcome of H. pylori infection.

Over the years, the understanding of H. pylori and its implications for human health has led to significant advancements in medical research, diagnostics, and treatment strategies. Researchers and healthcare professionals continue to study H. pylori to better understand its biology, how it causes diseases, and how to effectively manage and treat infections to improve the overall health and well-being of individuals affected by this bacterium.

1.2 Historical Perspective

The history of Helicobacter pylori (H. pylori) and its discovery is a fascinating journey that has revolutionized our understanding of peptic ulcers and gastric diseases. Prior to the discovery of H. pylori's role in these conditions, medical knowledge about ulcers and gastritis was quite different.

Early Beliefs and Misconceptions:

- **Ancient Theories:**
  Historically, peptic ulcers and gastritis were often attributed to factors such as stress, spicy foods, and an overproduction of stomach acid. These beliefs persisted for centuries.

- **Surgical Interventions:** In the 19th and early 20th centuries, surgical treatments, like gastrectomy (removal of part or all of the stomach), were considered for ulcers, reflecting the limited understanding of the underlying causes.

Barry Marshall and Robin Warren:

- The breakthrough in understanding the true cause of these conditions came in the early 1980s. Australian scientists Dr. Barry Marshall

and Dr. Robin Warren
challenged prevailing medical
wisdom by suggesting that
bacteria, specifically H. pylori,
might be responsible for
gastritis and ulcers.

- In 1982, they conducted a
  groundbreaking study in which
  they isolated H. pylori from the
  stomach lining of patients with
  gastritis and ulcers. This
  discovery was met with
  skepticism initially, as it
  contradicted established
  medical dogma.

- To prove their hypothesis,
  Barry Marshall even drank a
  culture of H. pylori to
  intentionally infect himself,
  leading to the development of
  gastritis. This act of self-
  experimentation ultimately

demonstrated the bacterium's ability to cause disease.

- In recognition of their groundbreaking work, Barry Marshall and Robin Warren were awarded the Nobel Prize in Physiology or Medicine in 2005.

Paradigm Shift and Medical Impact:

- The discovery of H. pylori marked a paradigm shift in the field of gastroenterology. It challenged conventional thinking about ulcers and gastritis and opened new avenues for understanding and treating these conditions.

- With the recognition of H. pylori's role, the focus of treatment shifted from merely addressing symptoms with antacids to targeting the underlying bacterial infection. This led to the development of effective antibiotic therapies.

- The discovery also had a profound impact on public health, as it reduced the need for unnecessary surgeries and provided more targeted treatment options for patients with ulcers and gastritis.

Ongoing Research and Implications:

- Since its discovery, research into H. pylori has continued to expand. Scientists have delved into its genetics, virulence factors, and mechanisms of infection.

- Studies have revealed associations between H. pylori and various gastrointestinal diseases, including stomach cancer, highlighting the importance of early detection and treatment.

- Ongoing research aims to understand the complex interactions between H. pylori, host genetics, and environmental factors in disease development, paving the way for personalized treatment approaches.

In summary, the historical perspective of H. pylori underscores the transformative impact of scientific discovery on medical practice. The identification of this bacterium challenged long-held beliefs, improved patient care, and continues to drive research aimed at better understanding and managing gastrointestinal diseases.

1.3 Why is H. pylori Important?

Helicobacter pylori (H. pylori) is of paramount importance in the fields of medicine and gastroenterology for several compelling reasons:

1. Major Cause of Gastric Diseases:

- H. pylori is a leading cause of various gastrointestinal diseases, including gastritis, peptic ulcers, and gastric cancer. These conditions can significantly impact an individual's quality of life and, in the case of cancer, be life-threatening. Understanding and managing H. pylori infection is critical in preventing and treating these diseases.

2. Paradigm Shift in Medical Understanding:

- The discovery of H. pylori's role in gastric diseases marked a paradigm shift in medical thinking. Prior to its recognition, ulcers and gastritis were often attributed to factors like stress and excessive stomach acid production. The discovery of H. pylori challenged these beliefs and led to more accurate diagnoses and effective treatments.

3. Reducing Unnecessary Surgeries:

- H. pylori's discovery and the subsequent understanding of its role in ulcers and gastritis significantly reduced the need for unnecessary surgical interventions. In the past, some patients underwent gastric surgery, including partial or total gastrectomy, to treat what was thought to be untreatable conditions. Recognizing H. pylori as a treatable cause has spared many patients from such invasive procedures.

4. Antibiotic Treatment Options:

- The identification of H. pylori as a bacterial infection led to the development of targeted antibiotic therapies. Prior to this discovery, treatment options for ulcers and gastritis were primarily focused on symptom relief, such as antacids. Antibiotic treatment regimens have proven highly effective in eradicating the bacterium and resolving associated conditions.

5. Reduced Disease Burden:

- Successful treatment of H. pylori infection has contributed to a reduction in the incidence of peptic ulcers and associated complications. This has led to improved patient outcomes and a decrease in the economic burden associated with managing these chronic conditions.

6. Link to Gastric Cancer Prevention:

- H. pylori infection is a significant risk factor for the development of gastric (stomach) cancer. By identifying and treating H.

pylori infections, especially in
high-risk populations, it is
possible to reduce the incidence
of gastric cancer. This has
important implications for
cancer prevention and early
detection efforts.

7. Ongoing Research Opportunities:

- H. pylori continues to be a
  subject of extensive research.
  Scientists study its genetics,
  virulence factors, and
  interactions with the human
  immune system. This ongoing
  research provides insights into
  the bacterium's mechanisms of
  infection and informs the
  development of new diagnostic
  tools and treatment strategies.

8. Public Health Impact:

- On a broader scale, the recognition of H. pylori's importance has had a positive impact on public health. Improved understanding of its role in disease has led to public health campaigns and educational efforts aimed at raising awareness about risk factors, symptoms, and the importance of early diagnosis and treatment.

H. pylori is important because it plays a central role in the development of gastrointestinal diseases, its discovery transformed medical understanding and treatment approaches, and its management has led to improved patient outcomes and a reduced burden of associated conditions. Additionally, ongoing research into H. pylori offers the potential for

further advancements in
gastroenterology and public health.

CHAPTER 2

Understanding H. pylori Infection

2.1 Transmission and Spread

Understanding how Helicobacter pylori (H. pylori) is transmitted and spreads is essential for preventing new infections and managing existing ones. H. pylori is primarily a human pathogen that colonizes the stomach and upper part of the small intestine. Here's a closer look at how this bacterium is transmitted and spreads:

1. Person-to-Person Transmission:

- The most common mode of H. pylori transmission is from

person to person. It typically occurs through close personal contact, especially within families. Factors that contribute to person-to-person transmission include sharing eating utensils, food, and drinks. Saliva may also contain the bacterium, making kissing a potential route of transmission.

2. Fecal-Oral Transmission:

- Another significant route of transmission is the fecal-oral route. H. pylori can be present in the feces of infected individuals. Poor hygiene practices, inadequate handwashing, or contamination of water and food sources with fecal matter can lead to the ingestion of the bacterium, thereby facilitating its spread.

3. Contaminated Water and Food:

- Contaminated water and food sources can serve as vehicles for H. pylori transmission. In areas with limited access to clean drinking water and poor sanitation facilities, there is an increased risk of H. pylori infection through the consumption of contaminated water or food, such as raw or undercooked shellfish, vegetables, or fruits irrigated with contaminated water.

4. Oral-to-Oral Transmission:

- H. pylori has been found in dental plaque and the oral cavity of infected individuals. There is evidence to suggest that the oral route may also play a role in transmission, although it is less common than fecal-oral or person-to-person transmission.

5. Childhood Infections:

- H. pylori infections often occur during childhood and tend to persist into adulthood if left untreated. Transmission in childhood can result from close contact with infected family members, especially parents or caregivers.

6. Environmental Factors:

- Environmental factors, such as living conditions, sanitation practices, and access to clean water, can influence the prevalence of H. pylori in a population. In areas with crowded living conditions and limited sanitation infrastructure, the risk of transmission may be higher.

7. Genetic Susceptibility:

- While transmission routes are crucial, not everyone exposed to H. pylori becomes infected. Genetic factors and individual immune responses play a role in susceptibility to infection and the development of associated diseases.

8. Reinfection:

- After successful treatment of H. pylori infection, there is a risk of reinfection, especially in environments with a high prevalence of the bacterium. Reinfection can occur through the same transmission routes as primary infection.

Understanding how H. pylori is transmitted and spreads highlights the importance of hygiene practices, clean drinking water, and public health measures to reduce the incidence of new infections. Additionally, recognizing transmission routes informs strategies for the management and prevention of H. pylori-related diseases, such as peptic ulcers and gastric cancer. Early detection and appropriate treatment of infections can also help reduce the spread of this bacterium within communities.

2.2 Symptoms and Complications of H. pylori Infection

Helicobacter pylori (H. pylori) infection can manifest with a range of symptoms and potential complications. However, it's important to note that many individuals infected with H. pylori may remain asymptomatic for years or even decades. Symptoms, when they do occur, can vary in severity. Here's an overview of the symptoms and potential complications associated with H. pylori infection:

Common Symptoms:

1. **Gastritis:** Inflammation of the stomach lining (gastritis) is a common outcome of H. pylori infection. Gastritis can lead to various symptoms, including:

    - **Abdominal pain or discomfort:** Often described as a burning or gnawing sensation in the upper abdomen.

- **Nausea and vomiting:** Some individuals may experience nausea or occasional vomiting.

- **Bloating:** Abdominal bloating and discomfort may be present.

- **Loss of appetite:** A reduced desire to eat may occur due to discomfort.

2. **Peptic Ulcers:** H. pylori is a major risk factor for the development of peptic ulcers. Symptoms of peptic ulcers can include:

   - **Burning or gnawing pain:** Similar to gastritis, peptic ulcers often cause a burning or gnawing pain in the upper abdomen, typically

between meals or at
night.

- **Indigestion:** Symptoms
may include bloating,
belching, and a feeling of
fullness.

- **Nausea and vomiting:**
These symptoms may be
more severe in the case
of ulcers.

Less Common Symptoms: 3.
**Gastroesophageal Reflux Disease
(GERD):** Some individuals with H.
pylori infection may experience
symptoms of GERD, including
heartburn, regurgitation, and difficulty
swallowing.

4. **Unexplained Weight Loss:** In
some cases, unexplained weight
loss can occur as a result of
reduced appetite and digestive

discomfort associated with H.
pylori infection.

5. **Iron Deficiency Anemia:**
Chronic H. pylori infection can
lead to iron deficiency anemia
due to impaired absorption of
iron in the stomach.

Complications:

1. **Peptic Ulcer Complications:**
Untreated peptic ulcers can lead
to serious complications, such
as:

   - **Bleeding Ulcers:** Ulcers
     can erode blood vessels,
     leading to
     gastrointestinal bleeding.
     This can result in
     symptoms like bloody
     vomit or dark, tarry
     stools.

- **Perforation:** In rare cases, ulcers may penetrate the stomach or duodenal wall, causing a perforation, a medical emergency that requires immediate surgery.

- **Obstruction:** Scarring from chronic ulcers can cause narrowing of the digestive tract, leading to a blockage (obstruction) and associated symptoms like vomiting and severe abdominal pain.

2. **Gastric Cancer:** Long-term H. pylori infection is a significant risk factor for the development of gastric (stomach) cancer. It is one of the leading causes of gastric cancer worldwide. Most individuals with H. pylori

infection do not develop cancer, but the presence of the bacterium increases the risk, especially in those with certain genetic predispositions.

3. **MALT Lymphoma:** In rare cases, H. pylori infection can lead to the development of MALT (mucosa-associated lymphoid tissue) lymphoma, a type of non-Hodgkin lymphoma that affects the stomach lining.

It's important to emphasize that not everyone with H. pylori infection will experience symptoms or complications. In fact, a significant portion of infected individuals remains asymptomatic. Additionally, prompt diagnosis and appropriate treatment can help alleviate symptoms and reduce the risk of complications associated with H. pylori infection. If you suspect an H. pylori infection or experience persistent gastrointestinal symptoms, it's advisable to seek medical evaluation and guidance for proper diagnosis and management.

2.3 Diagnosis of H. pylori Infection

Diagnosing Helicobacter pylori (H. pylori) infection is crucial for determining whether an individual has the bacterium and whether treatment is necessary. Several diagnostic methods are available, each with its own advantages and limitations. Here are some of the common approaches to diagnosing H. pylori infection:

1. **Urea Breath Test:**

- The urea breath test is a non-invasive and highly accurate method for detecting H. pylori. It involves the ingestion of a special urea solution that contains a harmless, labeled form of carbon. If H. pylori is present in the stomach, it produces an enzyme called urease, which breaks down the urea and releases labeled carbon dioxide. The patient exhales into a sample container, and the exhaled breath is tested for the presence of labeled carbon dioxide.

- This test is often preferred because it is non-invasive, does not require any special preparation, and provides rapid results.

2. Stool Antigen Test:

- In this test, a stool sample is collected and analyzed for the presence of H. pylori antigens, which are specific proteins produced by the bacterium. Stool antigen tests are non-invasive and are particularly useful for diagnosing H. pylori infection in children or when other methods are less suitable.

- This method is convenient for pediatric patients and those who may not tolerate other testing procedures.

3. **Blood Antibody Test:**

- Blood antibody tests measure the presence of antibodies against H. pylori in the bloodstream. When the body is exposed to H. pylori, it produces antibodies as part of

the immune response.
Detecting these antibodies can
indicate a current or past H.
pylori infection.

- While blood antibody tests are
  non-invasive, they have
  limitations. They cannot
  distinguish between current and
  past infections, and antibodies
  may persist in the blood even
  after successful treatment.

4. Upper Endoscopy (Esophagogastroduodenoscopy - EGD):

- An upper endoscopy is an
  invasive procedure in which a
  thin, flexible tube with a
  camera (endoscope) is inserted
  through the mouth and into the
  esophagus, stomach, and
  duodenum. During this

procedure, biopsies can be taken from the stomach lining to directly visualize and confirm the presence of H. pylori.

- Biopsy samples can be tested using various methods, including histology (microscopic examination), rapid urease testing, and culture.

5. **Biopsy-based Tests:**

- During an upper endoscopy, small tissue samples (biopsies) can be collected from the stomach lining. These biopsy samples can be tested using different techniques, including:

  - **Histology:** Microscopic examination of tissue

samples for the presence of H. pylori bacteria.

- **Rapid Urease Test:** A small piece of tissue is placed in a special test solution. If H. pylori is present, it produces urease, leading to a color change in the solution.

- **Culture:** H. pylori can be cultured (grown) from the biopsy samples in a laboratory.

6. PCR (Polymerase Chain Reaction):

- PCR is a molecular technique that can detect the genetic material (DNA) of H. pylori in clinical samples, such as biopsies or stool. It is a highly sensitive method that can provide accurate results.

The choice of diagnostic method may depend on factors such as the patient's age, medical history, symptoms, and the availability of specific tests at the healthcare facility. In some cases, healthcare providers may use a combination of tests to increase the accuracy of diagnosis. Once H. pylori infection is confirmed, appropriate treatment can be prescribed to eradicate the bacterium and manage associated conditions like gastritis and peptic ulcers.

CHAPTER 3

Causes and Risk Factors

3.1 How H. pylori Infection Occurs

Helicobacter pylori (H. pylori) infection occurs when individuals are exposed to and subsequently colonized by the bacterium. The exact mechanisms of transmission and infection are not fully understood, but several factors contribute to how H. pylori infection occurs:

1. Person-to-Person Contact:

- Close personal contact with an infected individual is a common route of transmission.

This includes family members, caregivers, and individuals who share eating utensils, food, or beverages with an infected person. Kissing, especially between family members or intimate partners, can also facilitate transmission.

2. Fecal-Oral Transmission:

- H. pylori can be found in the feces of infected individuals. Poor hygiene practices, inadequate handwashing, and the contamination of water and food sources with fecal matter can lead to the ingestion of H. pylori. This is known as the fecal-oral route of transmission.

3. Contaminated Water and Food:

- In regions with limited access to clean drinking water and inadequate sanitation facilities, there is an increased risk of H. pylori transmission through the consumption of contaminated water or food. This can include drinking water contaminated with sewage or consuming raw or undercooked seafood, vegetables, or fruits irrigated with contaminated water.

4. Childhood Infections:

- H. pylori infections often begin in childhood. Children are more susceptible to infection, possibly due to factors such as immune system immaturity and close contact with infected family members or caregivers.

5. Oral Route:

- There is evidence to suggest that H. pylori can also be

transmitted through the oral route. The bacterium can be present in dental plaque and the oral cavity of infected individuals. It is possible that oral-oral transmission may occur through activities like sharing utensils or engaging in close contact, but this route is less common than fecal-oral or person-to-person transmission.

6. Environmental Factors:

- Living conditions and environmental factors can influence the prevalence of H. pylori in a population. Crowded living conditions, limited access to clean water, and poor sanitation infrastructure can contribute to the higher prevalence of H. pylori in certain areas.

7. Genetic Susceptibility:

- Not everyone exposed to H. pylori becomes infected, and individuals' genetic factors may influence their susceptibility to infection. Some people may have genetic traits that make them more or less likely to acquire H. pylori.

8. Reinfection:

- After successful treatment of H. pylori infection, there is a risk of reinfection, especially in areas with a high prevalence of the bacterium. Reinfection can occur through the same transmission routes as primary infection.

It's important to note that while H. pylori infection is common worldwide, not all individuals who are exposed to the bacterium will develop symptoms or complications. The interplay between host factors (such as genetics and immune responses), environmental factors, and the specific strain of H. pylori can influence the outcome of infection. Additionally, H. pylori infections can be asymptomatic for many years, making early detection and treatment important for those at risk of complications like peptic ulcers and gastric cancer.

3.2 Risk Factors for H. pylori Infection

Helicobacter pylori (H. pylori) infection is influenced by various risk factors, both individual and environmental. While H. pylori infection is prevalent worldwide, certain factors can increase an individual's likelihood of becoming infected. Here are common risk factors associated with H. pylori infection:

1. Geographic Location:

- H. pylori infection rates vary significantly by geographical region. Infection is more common in developing countries and areas with lower socioeconomic status. Regions with a higher prevalence of H. pylori include parts of Africa, Asia, and South America.

2. Age:

- H. pylori infection often occurs during childhood. Younger individuals, especially children, are more susceptible to initial infection, possibly due to differences in immune responses. The risk of infection decreases with age.

3. Household Contact:

- Close contact with family members or caregivers who are infected with H. pylori can increase the risk of transmission. Sharing eating utensils, food, and close personal contact, such as kissing, can facilitate the spread of the bacterium within households.

4. Poor Sanitation and Hygiene:

- Inadequate access to clean drinking water and poor sanitation facilities can contribute to H. pylori transmission. Contaminated water and poor hygiene practices can result in the ingestion of the bacterium, particularly through the fecal-oral route.

5. Socioeconomic Status:

- Individuals with lower socioeconomic status may have a higher risk of H. pylori infection. This is often related to factors such as crowded living conditions, limited access to healthcare, and reduced access to clean water and sanitation facilities.

6. Childhood Environment:

- Early-life exposure to H. pylori is a significant risk factor. Children who grow up in households with infected individuals are more likely to acquire the infection themselves. Childhood infections tend to persist into adulthood if left untreated.

7. Crowded Living Conditions:

- Crowded living conditions, such as in densely populated urban areas or communal living environments, can facilitate the transmission of H. pylori among individuals.

8. Eating and Drinking Habits:

- Consumption of contaminated water or food, especially raw or undercooked seafood, vegetables, or fruits irrigated with contaminated water, can increase the risk of H. pylori infection. Individuals with these dietary habits may be at higher risk in areas with a higher prevalence of the bacterium.

9. Genetic Factors:

- Host genetics can play a role in susceptibility to H. pylori infection. Some individuals may have genetic traits that make them more or less prone to acquiring and retaining the bacterium.

10. Reinfection:

- Individuals who have previously been treated for H. pylori infection are at risk of reinfection, especially if they are exposed to the bacterium again through close contact or contaminated sources.

11. Immune System Function:

- Immune responses can vary among individuals, affecting their ability to clear H. pylori infections. A weakened immune system may be less effective in controlling or eliminating the bacterium.

It's important to note that while these risk factors are associated with H. pylori infection, not everyone with these risk factors will become infected, and conversely, individuals without these risk factors can still acquire the infection. The interplay between individual susceptibility, environmental factors, and the prevalence of H. pylori in a given region determines an individual's risk of infection. Early detection and appropriate treatment are essential for those at risk of developing complications like gastritis, peptic ulcers, or gastric cancer.

CHAPTER 4

H. pylori Testing and Diagnosis

4.1 Methods of Detection

Detecting Helicobacter pylori (H. pylori) infection is crucial for diagnosing associated gastrointestinal conditions and determining the need for treatment. There are several methods for detecting H. pylori, each with its own advantages and limitations. The choice of method may depend on factors such as the patient's age, symptoms, medical history, and available resources. Here are common methods of H. pylori detection:

1. **Urea Breath Test:**

- The urea breath test is a non-invasive and highly accurate method for detecting H. pylori. It involves the ingestion of a special urea solution that contains a harmless, labeled form of carbon. If H. pylori is present in the stomach, it produces an enzyme called urease, which breaks down the urea and releases labeled carbon dioxide. The patient exhales into a sample container, and the exhaled breath is tested for the presence of labeled carbon dioxide.

- This test is often preferred because it is non-invasive, does not require any special preparation, and provides rapid results.

2. Stool Antigen Test:

- In this test, a stool sample is collected and analyzed for the presence of H. pylori antigens, which are specific proteins produced by the bacterium. Stool antigen tests are non-invasive and are particularly useful for diagnosing H. pylori infection in children or when other methods are less suitable.

- This method is convenient for pediatric patients and those who may not tolerate other testing procedures.

3. **Blood Antibody Test:**

- Blood antibody tests measure the presence of antibodies against H. pylori in the bloodstream. When the body is exposed to H. pylori, it produces antibodies as part of

the immune response.
Detecting these antibodies can
indicate a current or past H.
pylori infection.

- While blood antibody tests are
  non-invasive, they have
  limitations. They cannot
  distinguish between current and
  past infections, and antibodies
  may persist in the blood even
  after successful treatment.

4. Upper Endoscopy (Esophagogastroduodenoscopy - EGD):

- An upper endoscopy is an
  invasive procedure in which a
  thin, flexible tube with a
  camera (endoscope) is inserted
  through the mouth and into the
  esophagus, stomach, and
  duodenum. During this

procedure, biopsies can be taken from the stomach lining to directly visualize and confirm the presence of H. pylori.

- Biopsy samples can be tested using various methods, including histology (microscopic examination), rapid urease testing, and culture.

5. Biopsy-based Tests:

- During an upper endoscopy, small tissue samples (biopsies) can be collected from the stomach lining. These biopsy samples can be tested using different techniques, including:

  - **Histology:** Microscopic examination of tissue samples

for the presence of H. pylori bacteria.

- **Rapid Urease Test:** A small piece of tissue is placed in a special test solution. If H. pylori is present, it produces urease, leading to a color change in the solution.

- **Culture:** H. pylori can be cultured (grown) from the biopsy samples in a laboratory.

6. PCR (Polymerase Chain Reaction):

- PCR is a molecular technique that can detect the genetic material (DNA) of H. pylori in clinical samples, such as biopsies or stool. It is a highly sensitive method that can provide accurate results.

The choice of diagnostic method may depend on factors such as the patient's age, medical history, symptoms, and the availability of specific tests at the healthcare facility. In some cases, healthcare providers may use a combination of tests to increase the accuracy of diagnosis.

4.2 When to Seek Testing

Seeking Helicobacter pylori (H. pylori) testing is important in various situations, especially when individuals have specific risk factors, symptoms, or medical conditions. Here are some scenarios in which individuals should consider seeking H. pylori testing:

1. Gastrointestinal Symptoms:

- Individuals experiencing persistent gastrointestinal symptoms should consider H. pylori testing. Common symptoms include:

    - **Stomach pain or discomfort:** Including a burning or gnawing sensation in the upper abdomen.

    - **Nausea and vomiting:** Especially if these symptoms persist.

    - **Bloating and fullness:** Particularly after meals.

    - **Indigestion:** Including symptoms like belching and a feeling of fullness.

2. Peptic Ulcer Symptoms:

- Peptic ulcers are a well-known complication of H. pylori infection. Seek testing if you experience symptoms of peptic ulcers, which can include:

- **Burning or gnawing abdominal pain:** Typically between meals or at night.

- **Nausea and vomiting:** Especially if associated with blood.

- **Dark, tarry stools or bloody vomit:** Indicative of bleeding ulcers.

3. Previous H. pylori Treatment:

- If you have been previously treated for H. pylori infection, testing may be recommended to confirm eradication of the bacterium. A follow-up test after treatment is important to ensure that the infection has been successfully eliminated.

4. Family or Household Exposure:

- If you have close family members or household contacts who have been diagnosed with H. pylori infection, you may have an increased risk of exposure and should consider testing, especially if you experience symptoms.

5. Family History of Gastric Cancer:

- Individuals with a family history of gastric (stomach) cancer may have an increased risk of H. pylori infection. Testing for H. pylori can be important for early detection and prevention efforts.

6. Iron Deficiency Anemia:

- Chronic H. pylori infection can lead to iron deficiency anemia due to impaired iron absorption. If you have unexplained iron deficiency anemia, your healthcare provider may recommend testing for H. pylori.

7. Prior or Current Gastric Cancer or MALT Lymphoma:

- Individuals with a history of gastric cancer or mucosa-associated lymphoid tissue (MALT) lymphoma may have had H. pylori infection as a contributing factor. Testing may be necessary for ongoing monitoring and treatment decisions.

8. Dyspepsia:

- In cases of unexplained dyspepsia (chronic or recurrent discomfort or pain in the upper abdomen), especially in adults under 60 years of age, H. pylori testing may be considered.

9. Persistent H. pylori Risk Factors:

- If you have ongoing risk factors for H. pylori exposure, such as living in an area with a high prevalence of the bacterium or having poor hygiene practices, regular testing may be recommended.

It's important to consult with a healthcare provider for appropriate evaluation and guidance if you suspect H. pylori infection or if you have risk factors or symptoms that warrant testing. Early diagnosis and treatment of H. pylori infection can help manage associated conditions, prevent complications, and improve overall health and quality of life. The choice of testing method will depend on individual circumstances and medical recommendations.

CHAPTER 5

Treatment Options

5.1 Antibiotics and Medications

Helicobacter pylori (H. pylori) infection is typically treated with a combination of antibiotics and medications. The primary goal of treatment is to eradicate the bacterium, which can help alleviate symptoms, heal the associated gastritis or peptic ulcers, and reduce the risk of complications. Here are the key components of H. pylori treatment:

1. Antibiotics:

- Antibiotics are the cornerstone of H. pylori treatment. A combination of antibiotics is often prescribed to target and eradicate the bacterium effectively. Commonly used antibiotics include:

  - **Clarithromycin**

  - **Amoxicillin**

  - **Metronidazole**

  - **Tetracycline**

- The specific antibiotic regimen may vary based on factors such as regional antibiotic resistance patterns and individual patient characteristics. Your healthcare provider will determine the most appropriate antibiotic combination for your case.

2. Proton Pump Inhibitors (PPIs):

- Proton pump inhibitors, such as omeprazole, lansoprazole, or esomeprazole, are medications that reduce stomach acid production. They are often prescribed alongside antibiotics to create an environment in which H. pylori is less able to thrive.

- PPIs help relieve symptoms and promote healing of gastritis and ulcers. They are typically taken for a period of 10 to 14 days in combination with antibiotics.

3. Bismuth Subsalicylate:

- Bismuth subsalicylate is another medication that may be included in the treatment regimen. It has antimicrobial properties and can help reduce H. pylori colonization in the

stomach. Bismuth subsalicylate
is available in various over-the-
counter formulations.

4. Follow-Up Testing:

- After completing the antibiotic
  and medication regimen,
  follow-up testing is essential to
  confirm the eradication of H.
  pylori. This is typically done
  several weeks after treatment
  completion to ensure that the
  infection has been successfully
  eliminated.

5. Treatment Challenges:

- H. pylori treatment can be
  challenging due to the
  development of antibiotic
  resistance. Some strains of H.
  pylori have become resistant to
  one or more antibiotics, making
  eradication more difficult. In

such cases, alternative antibiotic regimens may be necessary.

5.2 Lifestyle Changes

In addition to antibiotic treatment and medications, lifestyle changes can play a supportive role in managing H. pylori infection and reducing the risk of complications. Here are some lifestyle modifications that may be recommended:

1. Dietary Adjustments:

- While dietary changes cannot eradicate H. pylori on their own, they can help reduce symptoms and support healing. Recommendations may include:

- Avoiding spicy or acidic foods that can irritate the stomach lining.

- Limiting or avoiding alcohol and caffeine, which can increase stomach acid production.

- Eating smaller, more frequent meals to reduce stomach discomfort.

2. Smoking Cessation:

- Smoking can exacerbate gastritis and peptic ulcers, so quitting smoking is advisable. Smoking can also increase the risk of developing complications from H. pylori infection, such as gastric cancer.

3. Stress Management:

- High levels of stress can contribute to gastrointestinal symptoms. Practicing stress-reduction techniques, such as mindfulness, meditation, or yoga, may help improve overall well-being.

4. Hydration:

- Staying well-hydrated is important, especially during and after H. pylori treatment. Adequate hydration can help support healing and overall digestive health.

5. Follow Medical Advice:

- It's essential to follow your healthcare provider's instructions and complete the full course of antibiotics and medications as prescribed. Skipping doses or stopping

treatment prematurely can lead
to treatment failure or the
development of antibiotic
resistance.

6. Regular Follow-Up:

- After successful H. pylori
  treatment, regular follow-up
  appointments with your
  healthcare provider are
  important to monitor your
  progress and address any
  ongoing symptoms or concerns.

H. pylori treatment is effective in the
majority of cases, and it is essential to
complete the prescribed regimen and
follow medical advice to ensure
successful eradication of the
bacterium. Lifestyle changes can help
alleviate symptoms and support
healing but should be done in
conjunction with medical treatment

and guidance. If you have H. pylori infection or suspect you may have it, consult with a healthcare provider for an accurate diagnosis and appropriate treatment plan.

5.3 Alternative and Natural Remedies

While antibiotic treatment and medications prescribed by healthcare providers are the primary methods for eradicating Helicobacter pylori (H. pylori) infection, some individuals may be interested in complementary or natural remedies to support their overall gastrointestinal health or manage symptoms. It's essential to note that these alternative approaches are not a substitute for medical treatment, and consulting with a healthcare provider is crucial for proper diagnosis and treatment. Here are some alternative and natural remedies that have been explored:

1. Probiotics:

- Probiotics are beneficial bacteria that can help promote a healthy gut microbiome. Some studies suggest that certain probiotic strains may have a positive impact on H. pylori infection, such as Lactobacillus and Bifidobacterium species. However, more research is needed to confirm their effectiveness.

2. Manuka Honey:

- Manuka honey, derived from the nectar of the Manuka tree in New Zealand, has antimicrobial properties and may help inhibit the growth of H. pylori. It can be consumed as part of a balanced diet.

3. Cranberry Juice:

- Cranberry juice contains compounds that may help inhibit the adhesion of H. pylori to the stomach lining. Drinking pure, unsweetened cranberry juice in moderation may be a natural way to support digestive health.

4. Green Tea:

- Green tea contains antioxidants and compounds like catechins, which have been studied for their potential antimicrobial properties. Some research suggests that green tea extracts may have an inhibitory effect on H. pylori. Drinking green tea in moderation is generally considered safe and may offer other health benefits as well.

5. Garlic:

- Garlic contains a compound called allicin, which has antimicrobial properties. Some studies have explored the potential of garlic extracts or supplements in inhibiting H. pylori growth. Incorporating garlic into your diet may have other health benefits too.

6. Broccoli Sprouts:

- Broccoli sprouts contain a compound called sulforaphane, which has shown potential in laboratory studies for its ability to inhibit H. pylori growth. Consuming broccoli sprouts as part of a balanced diet may be a healthy addition.

7. Mastic Gum:

- Mastic gum is a resin extracted from the mastic tree, and it has been studied for its potential to inhibit H. pylori growth. Some individuals use mastic gum supplements, but its effectiveness varies among individuals.

8. Deglycyrrhizinated Licorice (DGL):

- DGL is a form of licorice that has had the compound glycyrrhizin removed to reduce its potential side effects. Some people use DGL supplements to help manage gastrointestinal symptoms, including those related to H. pylori infection.

9. Dietary Modifications:

- Adopting a balanced diet that includes fiber-rich foods, lean proteins, and fresh fruits and vegetables can promote overall digestive health. Avoiding spicy, acidic, and fatty foods may help reduce discomfort.

It's important to approach these alternative and natural remedies with caution and consult with a healthcare provider before using them, especially if you have an H. pylori infection. These remedies are not a substitute for prescribed antibiotics and medications, which are the most effective way to eradicate the bacterium. Additionally, some natural remedies may interact with medications or have side effects, so it's essential to discuss their use with a healthcare professional.

CHAPTER 6

Managing H. pylori Infection

Helicobacter pylori (H. pylori) infection can be effectively managed with appropriate treatment and lifestyle adjustments. Recovery and preventing recurrence are important aspects of managing this infection. Here are some tips and strategies for managing H. pylori infection:

6.1 Tips for Recovery

1. **Follow Medical Treatment:** If you have been diagnosed with H. pylori infection, follow your healthcare provider's prescribed

treatment regimen diligently. Take all antibiotics and medications as directed, and complete the full course of treatment, even if you start feeling better before finishing.

2. **Take Medications as Prescribed:** If you have been prescribed medications such as proton pump inhibitors (PPIs) or bismuth subsalicylate along with antibiotics, take them according to your provider's instructions. These medications help reduce stomach acid and create a favorable environment for antibiotic efficacy.

3. **Stay Hydrated:** Adequate hydration is essential during and after treatment. It helps support the healing of the

stomach lining and overall digestive health.

4. **Monitor Symptoms:** Pay attention to your symptoms during and after treatment. If you experience persistent or worsening symptoms or side effects from medications, contact your healthcare provider promptly.

5. **Follow-Up Testing:** After completing treatment, schedule follow-up testing as recommended by your healthcare provider. This is crucial to confirm that the infection has been successfully eradicated.

6. **Manage Stress:** High levels of stress can exacerbate gastrointestinal symptoms.

Consider stress-reduction techniques such as mindfulness, meditation, yoga, or counseling to help manage stress and improve overall well-being.

7. **Dietary Adjustments:** While diet alone cannot eliminate H. pylori infection, making dietary changes can help reduce symptoms and support healing. Avoid spicy, acidic, and fatty foods that can irritate the stomach lining. Instead, opt for a balanced diet rich in fiber, lean proteins, and fresh fruits and vegetables.

6.2 Preventing Recurrence

1. **Practice Good Hygiene:** To reduce the risk of reinfection, practice good hygiene, including regular handwashing with soap and water, especially before eating. Avoid sharing eating utensils, food, or beverages with individuals who may be infected.

2. **Maintain a Healthy Lifestyle:** Adopting a healthy lifestyle can help prevent H. pylori recurrence and promote overall digestive health. This includes:

   - Quitting smoking if you are a smoker.

   - Limiting alcohol consumption.

- Staying physically active.

- Managing your weight through a balanced diet and regular exercise.

3. **Avoid NSAIDs and Irritants:** Nonsteroidal anti-inflammatory drugs (NSAIDs) like aspirin and ibuprofen can irritate the stomach lining and increase the risk of complications. If you need to use NSAIDs, discuss alternatives with your healthcare provider.

4. **Monitor Your Health:** Be proactive about your health and seek medical attention if you experience recurring symptoms or any concerning changes in your digestive health.

5. **Screening for Gastric Cancer:** If you have a family history of gastric (stomach) cancer or other risk factors, discuss with your healthcare provider the need for periodic screening and surveillance to detect potential complications early.

6. **Antibiotic Resistance:** In regions with high rates of antibiotic resistance, reinfection can be a concern. Be aware of the antibiotic resistance patterns in your area and discuss with your healthcare provider the best treatment options available.

Remember that successful management of H. pylori infection involves a combination of medical treatment, lifestyle adjustments, and preventive measures. Consult with

your healthcare provider for
personalized guidance on managing
and preventing H. pylori infection
based on your specific circumstances
and health needs.

CHAPTER 7

H. pylori and its Connection to Health

Helicobacter pylori (H. pylori) is a bacterium that can have a significant impact on an individual's health. It is associated with various gastrointestinal conditions and can influence overall well-being. Here are some key connections between H. pylori and health:

7.1 Link to Gastric Ulcers

Gastric ulcers, also known as stomach ulcers, are one of the most well-known health conditions associated with H. pylori infection.

These ulcers are open sores that form on the lining of the stomach or the upper part of the small intestine (duodenum). The connection between H. pylori and gastric ulcers is as follows:

- **Causative Role:** H. pylori infection is a significant factor in the development of gastric ulcers. The bacterium can colonize the stomach lining and weaken the protective mucous layer, making it more susceptible to damage from stomach acid. This can lead to the formation of ulcers.

- **Chronic Inflammation:** H. pylori infection often results in chronic inflammation of the stomach lining (gastritis). Over time, this inflammation can contribute to ulcer formation.

- **Treatment:** Successfully eradicating H. pylori through antibiotic treatment and medications can lead to ulcer healing and a reduced risk of ulcer recurrence.

7.2 Association with Other Diseases

Beyond gastric ulcers, H. pylori has been linked to several other health conditions and diseases. While these associations exist, the mechanisms and implications are not fully understood, and ongoing research is exploring these connections. Some of the associations include:

- **Gastric Cancer:** Long-term H. pylori infection is a known risk factor for **gastric (stomach)**

cancer. The chronic inflammation caused by the bacterium can damage the stomach lining and increase the risk of cancerous changes over time. However, not everyone with H. pylori infection develops gastric cancer, and other factors, including genetics and environmental factors, play a role in cancer development.

- **Mucosa-Associated Lymphoid Tissue (MALT) Lymphoma:** H. pylori infection is associated with a rare type of lymphoma called **MALT lymphoma**. Successful treatment of the infection can lead to remission in some cases of MALT lymphoma.

- **Iron Deficiency Anemia:** Chronic H. pylori infection can lead to **iron deficiency anemia** due to impaired iron absorption in the stomach. Treating the infection may help improve iron levels in affected individuals.

- **Functional Dyspepsia:** Some individuals with H. pylori infection may experience **functional dyspepsia**, a condition characterized by chronic or recurrent upper abdominal discomfort or pain. Treatment may alleviate symptoms in some cases.

- **Reflux Esophagitis:** There is evidence to suggest that H. pylori infection may have a protective effect against **gastroesophageal reflux disease (GERD)** or reflux esophagitis. The bacterium may

reduce stomach acid
production, potentially leading
to fewer instances of acid
reflux.

It's important to note that not
everyone with H. pylori infection will
develop these associated health
conditions, and the risk varies among
individuals. Additionally, ongoing
research is providing more insights
into the complex relationship between
H. pylori and various diseases. For
individuals with H. pylori infection,
early diagnosis, appropriate treatment,
and regular follow-up with healthcare
providers are essential to manage
associated health risks and promote
overall well-being.